Losing weight Without a compulsory exercise

BEN WILLIAMS

ISBN: : 9781730728747

PREFACE

Exercise is a major key to most weight loss plans because it helps you burn more calories, the more calories you burn the more weight you lose. But what if you hate exercise? Is it required to lose weight? It certainly helps you stay healthier by revving your heart rate and building your muscles. But it is not compulsory. There are ways to lose pounds without exercising. Which I will be discussing in this book.

INTRODUCTION

Losing weight occurs when the body expends more calories than it consume. That means, the body have to burn off or eat fewer calories that you consume through meals and snacks. Many people reduce calories from their diet or burn calories through exercise in order to loss some pounds of weight. Working out on a regular basis is helpful while trying to lose weight, but may not be practical for some other people due to health conditions, time restraints, or lack of interest and focus. However, research shows that during weight loss struggle, diet plays a very unique role compared to exercise. It's more easier to reduce caloric intake by modifying your diet compared to burning off quality amount of calories through exercise. Making a few changes to your feeding method and lifestyle can help you lose weight safely and effectively without planed exercise.

TABLE OF CONTENT.

CHAPTER ONE

MODIFYING YOUR DIET WEIGHT LOSE.

CHAPTER TWO

MAINTAING YOUR WEIGHT LOSE.

- FIND A SUPPORTING GROUP.

- REWARD YOUR SELF.

CHAPTER THREE.

CHANGING YOUR LIFE STYLE FOR WEIGHT LOSE.

- START A FOOD JOURNAL

- GET ADEQUATE REST

- INCREASE YOUR BASELINE PHYSICAL ACTIVITIES

CHAPTER ONE

MODIFYING YOUR DIET WEIGHT LOSE.

COUNT CALORIES

Weight loss programs usually need you to modify your total calorie consumption. Counting calories and being aware of the quantity you consume will help you lose weight. In general, you'll like to cut out about 500–750 amount of calories in a day to lose about one to two pounds weekly.

Plan out how many calories you can cut from your daily consumptions by first calculating the amount of calories you should take in a day. Do these by searching the internet for a calorie calculator, then input your weight, height, age and activity level in order to calculate your recommended calories consumptions. People are different from one another, so it's better to get your own, personalized number.

Do not take in less than 1200 calories on a daily basis. A diet that's deficient in calories puts you at risk for nutrient deficiencies as you cannot eat the right amount of food to meet your daily requirements for most vitamins, minerals, and protein.

KNOW THE FACT THAT YOUR WEIGHT IS A BALANCING ACT

 Calorie intake is only a part of the equation. Fad diets may assure you that counting carbohydrates or consuming high amount of grapefruit will make the pounds reduce; but when it comes to weight loss, it's calories that matter. Weight loss comes down to burning higher amount of calories than you consume. You can do that by reducing extra amount of calories from food and beverages, and increase the rate of calories burning through physical activity.

EFFECTS OF OVERWEIGHT ON THE HUMAN BODY

In the year2003 statistics show that about one billion adults is considered to be obese, also in the year 2013 statistics show that there is a double increase in the number of obese as a result of careless method of our diet. This is another broad day enemy that is sending many people to an early grave, render them useless or making them look unattractive.

Excess weight is the un ideal weight that makes an individual look unhealthy, unattractive, ill relevant and unhappy especially among the female. one of the way that can make you look attractive and healthy is to maintain an ideal weight. If you must do this you need a diligent approach to achieve a better result.

Losing weight is not as easy or as quick as you may think, there are things you must do or there are sacrifices you must pay if you must achieve a good result such as avoiding some kind of foods for a healthier and attractive look. You must avoid some food that gives unnecessary fat like sugary cereal, its taste nice, yes I know it also looks attractive, yes I know but let me tell you they do more harm than good in the body system try as much as possible to put them out of your reach. Cereal is made from ultra-refined grain but cereal is high in calories and tends to be high in sugary, many cereals have as much sugar as a glazed donut.granted, calories wise, much high fiber cereals like fiber one is fairly low in energy, however, the more popular cereal that people that people actually eat are not low calories food. Cereal also activates brain chemical that makes you feel sedated. in often times we had misconception that cereal energizes your body system which is not always true, cereal stimulate an inhibitory system of transmitter in the brain, making the body system feel sedated and sleepy.incontrast food that is high in amino acids, such as quality protein stimulate the brain cells to keep you alert and vigilant. Cereal is so dangerous to body system because they have low-quality protein since it is made predominately from refined grains which are carbohydrate. However, there are many other foods that we can consume without exposing us to health threat such as protein in natural form.

Writing out a plan on how to excesses during the week and a meal plan, this helps greatly by committing yourself to achieve a good result. Eating healthy and exercise can seem like a pretty simple and straightforward goal, however, there are many different components to a healthy diet and fitness program. You need to choose a particular day of the week for walking out and also choose what food to eat, when to eat the food and how to prepare them. Starting with a specific goal and detail plan can help you implement the change you need you to need to help you eat healthier. Use food recall method to achieve this goal by planning what you eat and drink on a particular day in all your meals.

Always take your breakfast on regular basis, drink less soda and eat more vegetables. Eat enough vegetables and fruits because fruits and vegetables are of low calories and high in fibers, vitamins and minerals. it's also important you choose fruits and vegetable that are most nutrients dense. Physical activities are also of a great advantage to achieve a good result because through these process a certain amount of water and nutrient goes out of the body system through sweat. Such as gyms, swimming, dancing, hiking, walking etc.

Don't deprive yourself of any meal especially breakfast because breakfast is responsible for putting our metabolism in action for the day. The longer breakfast is delayed the longer it takes for metabolism to take place in order to burn fat in the body system, take light food as breakfast so as to start metabolism without overloading it with calories. Take more water with the low amount of calories such as sad because this can prevent several hundred of calories from going into the body system.

chew slowly whenever you are eating food and make sure all your food are finely mused not only does this in the digestive system but it makes you full easily, the reason for this is that if the food is chewed stay chunky through digestion and build up in the stomach area.

Eat slowly because it takes the brain up to 20 minutes to send a message to the system that you ate, so if slowly you are eating by the time you finished the message is sent and you will not eat an unnecessary extra serving.

WRITE YOURSELF A MEAL PLAN OR GUIDE

If you are not exercising to burn calories, you must trim them off from your diet in order to lose weight effectively. Writing out a meal plan or guide can help you plan out all your meals and snacks and make sure they blend into your pre-determined calorie range.

Spend some time writing out all your meals, snacks, and beverages for some days or a week.

Calculate a certain caloric amount for each meal. For such as: 300-calorie breakfast, two 500-calorie bigger meals, and one to two 100-calorie snacks. This will help you choose what foods to eat for meals and snacks throughout the day.

Include foods from all five food groups in some days. Review your meal plan or guide to make sure you're getting the right amounts of fruits, vegetables, whole grains, lean protein, and dairy.

Having all your meals and snacks planned in advance will

help you to avoid making poor nutrition choices when you're in a hurry.

Keep snacks conveniently located and ready in your fridge and car.

EAT A BALANCED DIET

Food that is calorie controlled and includes all five food groups is a good foundation for healthy weight loss. It's important You include all of the following most days:

Fruits and vegetables. These foods are loaded, filling, low-calorie and low-fat. Not only are fruits and veggies great for your waistline; they have ample amounts of vitamins, minerals, fiber, and antioxidants that you require for long-term health. Aim to make your meals to be more of fruits or vegetables.

Lean protein. Foods like poultry, eggs, pork, lean beef, legumes, dairy products, and tofu are great means of lean protein. Protein will keep you satisfied longer and may avoid hunger cravings. Include 3-4 of protein at every meal this is about the size of a deck of cards.

100% whole grains. Foods that are purely grains are high in fiber and some vitamins and minerals. Quinoa, oats, brown rice, millet, and 100% whole wheat pasta and bread are good examples of whole grains to include in your food. Limit your grains to 1/2 cup or 1 in a meal.

SNACK HEALTHY

 Putting one to two low-calorie snacks is proper when you're trying to lose weight. Many times a snack will assist your quest of weight loss.

Snacking may be good when there is more than five or six hours between your meals. Sometimes, going for long periods of time without eating may make it difficult for you to adhered to your planned meal or portion sizes as you may be overly hungry.

Most snacks included in a weight loss plan must be calorie controlled. Keep snacks between 100-200 calories.

EAT WITHOUT ELECTRONIC DISTRACTIONS

Paying attention to what you consume will help you consume lesser calories.

People who eat while they're watching television program or playing a computer games may take their mind off track of how much they have eaten. Which will lead to overeating? eating, eat about 10% more in that sitting.

If you regularly consume meals while watching TV or using electronic devices, you could be eating more unintentionally. These excess calories sum up and have a massive impact on your weight in the long term

KEEP UNHEALTHY FOODS OUT OF SIGHT

putting unhealthy foods where you can always see them may increase hunger and craves, that can make you to eat more which will lead to weight gain

One recent study shows that if high-calorie foods are easily accessible in the house, residents of that house are more likely to weigh more than people who keep only a bowl of fruit visible.

Keep unhealthy foods out of sight, such as in closets or cupboards, so that they will not easily catch your attention when you're hungry.

If you keep unhealthy foods on your counter, there will be tendency for you to have an unplanned method of eating.

CHEW THOROUGHLY AND SLOW DOWN

Your brain requires time to process that you've had enough to eat.

Grinding your food thoroughly makes you eat slowly, which will reduce the quantity of food intake, increased fullness and makes you to consume smaller portion.

How soon you finish your meals may also affect your weight negatively.

A recent findings show that faster eaters are more likely to gain weight than slower eaters.

People who eat very fast are also much more likely to be obese.

Eating more slowly, it may help to count how many times you chew each bite.

Eating your food slowly helps you feel full easily with fewer calories. It is an easy way to lose weight and prevent excess weight.

CHOOSE HEALTHIER COOKING TECHNIQUES.

 Don't corrupt your good intentions with bad preparation methods. Cooking methods that demand a lot of oil, butter, or other high-fat sauces or seasonings may cause your weight loss to plateau or slow.

Try cooking methods that don't demand much fat. Try steaming, grilling, roasting and poaching/boiling.

Adhered to extra virgin olive oil or canola oil. When substituted for saturated fats such as butter, these healthy single unsaturated fats can help to improve blood cholesterol levels, thereby reducing risk for heart disease and obesity or over weight.

Abstain from cooking techniques such as deep fat frying or pan frying. Also avoid cooking methods that demand a lot of butter, oil, or margarine.

DRINK ADEQUATE AMOUNTS OF FLUIDS.

Staying well-hydrated is also important to weight loss. Sometimes, thirst can feel similar to hunger and make you to eat. Drinking right require amount of fluid by the body can help prevent this mistake and promote weight loss.

Take up to 64 or about eight glasses of clear, sugar-free liquids every day. This is a generally recommended, but is a good place to begin.

Fluids that are useful in your daily goal include: water, sugar-free flavored waters, plain tea, and coffee without cream or sugar.

DITCH ALCOHOL AND SUGARY BEVERAGES.

Both alcoholic beverages and sugary beverages contain high amounts of calories that may contradict your weight loss plan. Ideally, completely pass these up as long as you want to continued weight loss.

Sugary beverages that you need to avoid include: regular soda, sweetened tea, sweetened coffee drinks, sports drinks and juices.

At most, women should consume one glass or less of alcohol on daily basis and men should consume two or less on daily basis also. Again, if continued weight loss is desired, alcohol should be avoided completely

CHAPTER TWO.
MAINTAINING YOUR WEIGHT LOSS

WEIGH YOURSELF ONCE OR TWICE A WEEK.

 Monitoring and read your progress is important when you're losing weight. Stepping on the scale most often can help you see how progress and effective your diet program is going and whether or not you need to make any changes or adhered to the initial plan.

It's important you know that, safe weight loss is about one to two pounds per week. Be patient and diligent with your progress. You're more likely to have a slow and steady weight loss in the long run.

For the most reliable pattern of results, it's best to weigh yourself at the same time on each day, on the same day of the week and in the same clothes (or choose to go without clothes).

If your weight loss has plateaue or you've started gaining weight, review your meal plans and food journals and see if you can reduce any more calories to help weight loss.

FIND A SUPPORT GROUP

Get friends, family members or co-workers that will be supporting you through your weight loss plan will help you continue to lose weight and maintain it long-term. Build a support group to help you remain focus.

Find out if others you know also want to lose weight. Most times people find it simpler to tackle weight loss together as a group.

You can as well find online support groups or support groups that meet in person either on weekly or monthly basis.

working with a registered dietitian will also help in making the task easier because he/she can customize your meal plan and provide on-going support.

REWARD YOURSELF

Having a motivating and enticing reward at the end of your weight loss struggle can help push you through to the end. Put aside something exciting for yourself as you meet your goals.

CHAPTER THREE

MAKING LIFESTYLE CHANGES FOR WEIGHT LOSS

START A FOOD JOURNAL

Journaling your meals, snacks and drinks will help encourage you to stay on track. Also, people who journal typically lose higher amount of weight and keep it off longer unlike to those who do not track their food.

You can purchase a journal or download a food journal app. Track as many days as possible. Also, you're more likely to remain on track and stick with your meal plan the more often you record your foods.

Keep track of your food journal. This may be a good resource to increase how well your diet is going and how effective it is for weight loss.

GET ADEQUATE REST

Having seven to nine hours sleep each night is recommended for general health and wellness. However, adequate sleep is also essential for weight loss. Research reveals that people who sleep less than six or seven hours nightly or poor sleep weigh more than those who get adequate rest.

Go to bed earlier. If you will like to get up early, try to get in bed earlier to meet the require sleeping hour. To ensure you have a sound and undisturbed sleep, remove all electronics garget like your phone, tablet device or computer from your bedroom.

Practice good sleeping habit to ensure you get the most out of your sleep.